W9-DFL-825

GET RID OF YOUR GUT

LOOK BETTER, FEEL BETTER, PREVENT BACK PAIN IN ONLY 64 MINUTES A WEEK

BY JEANETTE MICELOTTA, M.S., P.T.
AND DEBORAH MICHAELS, P.T.A.

INTRODUCTION BY DR. RICHARD BACHRACH
DIRECTOR, CENTER FOR SPORTS AND OSTEOPATHIC MEDICINE
PHOTOGRAPHS BY ELLEN WALLOP

A JOHN BOSWELL ASSOCIATES BOOK
HEARST BOOKS
NEW YORK

Copyright © 1993 by John Boswell Management, Inc.

All rights reserved. No part of this book may be reproduced or utilized in any form or by any means, electronic or mechanical, including photocopying, recording, or any information storage or retrieval system, without permission in writing from Publisher. Inquiries should be addressed to Permissions Department, William Morrow and Company, Inc., 1350 Avenue of the Americas, New York, N.Y. 10019.

It is the policy of William Morrow and Company, Inc., and its imprints and affiliates, recognizing the importance of preserving what has been written, to print the books we publish on acid-free paper, and we exert our best efforts to that end.

MODELS: Michael T. Brown
Claudia Porfilio

Library of Congress Cataloging-in-Publication Data
Micelotta, Jeanette.
    Get rid of your gut: look better, feel better, prevent back pain
    in only 64 minutes a week / Jeanette Micelotta, Deborah Michaels.
        p.   cm.
    ISBN 0-688-11886-0
        1. Abdominal exercises.   2. Backache—Prevention.
        I. Michaels, Deborah.   II. Title.
    RA781.M448   1993
    646.7'5—dc20   92-37813
                                                       CIP

Printed in the United States of America

    4   5   6   7   8   9   10

Book Design by Barbara Cohen Aronica

Contents

Introduction

By Richard Bachrach, D.O.

The Center for Sports and Osteopathic Medicine had its origin thirty-seven years ago, when I joined my father in the practice of osteopathic medicine. He jump-started my career by allowing me to learn musculoskeletal medicine through treating the many professional dancers in his practice. He had a problem with their care—he could not comprehend how anyone could be so motivated as to voluntarily commit himself or herself to the physical abuse demanded by the profession.

My father had a general aversion to physical activity of any sort. He espoused Ben Franklin's attitude: every time he felt the urge to exercise, he'd lie down until it passed. Forty to fifty years ago, active exercise was not regarded as part of the treatment protocol for low back pain (which constituted the bulk of our practice) by most other osteopathic physicians, "manipulators," or practitioners of manual medicine as well as by orthopedic surgeons.

But, by the standards of that time, we did quite well in the care of our back-pain patients. Or so we thought. Most of our patients got better, at least temporarily. The number of recurrences, however, was significant. As a matter of fact, the volume of our practice actually depended on so-called preventive maintenance therapy and on treatment of those recurrences.

Our patients were, in effect, addicted to our treatment and played an essentially passive role in their own care. They would return over and over for years. Many eventually had to resort to surgery to "cure" their back pain, but this too, in the long run, didn't work.

Slowly, with dancers, I recognized a deviation from the standard pattern. They didn't conform to the treatment plan. They resisted maintenance appointments and appeared to have fewer complaints referable to persistent or recurrent low back pain, although they certainly presented a diffuse array of other musculoskeletal ailments.

Gradually, the connection emerged. After many years of attending to their medical needs, I finally understood. Basically, it came down to flat tummies. Flat tummies happened with exercise. Dancers had less back pain and would respond more rapidly to treatment than the rest of my patient population, in spite of the tremendous stresses to which they subjected their bodies.

So began my sports-medicine approach to low back pain, which finally ovolvod into the Center for Sports and Osteopathic Medicine. Exercise, with emphasis on abdominal muscle strengthening, abdominal/pelvic stabilization, hip flexor (psoas) stretching, and low back strengthening has become the cornerstone of our program at the center.

The contributions of Jeanette Micelotta, our head physical therapist, and of Deborah Michaels, her chief assistant, have been essential to the development and success of this program. Through her extraordinary intelligence, remarkable clinical judgment, and exceptional leadership ability, Jeanette has provided the spark that drives it. Deborah has been instrumental in accurately and efficiently implementing Jeanette's programs and, at the same time, making her own innovative contributions. Together with the rest of our superbly talented staff, they have provided our patients with the tools to effectively self-manage their back care.

Our back-pain patients don't come to us looking for flat tummies, but for relief of pain and for functional restoration. The exercises designed by Jeanette and Deborah and presented in this excellent book are an essential part of our program. However, it's not just coincidental that our patients usually leave with those goals attained . . . and with flat tummies.

1

Get Rid of Your Gut

As both physical therapists and regular exercisers ourselves, we are great believers in the joys of sports, exercise, and physical activity, which is one of the reasons we experience so much satisfaction in helping our patients get back up to speed again. Exercise is extraordinary medicine and we see it work every day. Instead of having our patients take a pill every four hours, we give them specific exercises to perform. Through a combined twenty-eight years of professional experience as therapists, we know how the body is supposed to work and, when the muscles are weakened by pain or physical injury, we know what can be done to return the body to optimal performance.

Frankly, patients don't come to see us because they want to get rid of their gut. They come because they are experiencing physical discomfort of one form or another. The majority of our patients come to us with low back pain and, since strong abdominal muscles are essential to full recovery, they leave with the beneficial "side effect" of having a flatter and tighter midsection.

We treat a wide variety of patients of all ages, from dancers, athletes, actors, and authors, to corporate executives, lawyers, and accountants, and it is not surprising that back pain is the number-one reason for their visit. Indeed, 80 percent of all Americans will suffer low back pain at some point in their lives. These backaches cause more lost work time than any other physical ailment in this country, second overall only to the common cold. Back pain may be caused by a number of underlying problems, such as arthritis, tension and stress, bone spurs, or a jarring accident. Yet studies confirm that 90 percent of all low back pain is caused by muscular problems related to poor posture, a sedentary life-style, obesity—all symptoms or causes of weak stomach muscles.

Many people in New York City, where we work, develop back pain because of the demands of their jobs. The pace and stress level alone are enough to trigger back problems. Add to this typical business postures—slumped over a desk, slouched in an office chair, cradling the phone for hours at a time—and it's a wonder that incidences of back pain are as "low" as 80 percent.

Through our work with patients at the Center for Sports and Osteopathic Medicine, we have found that the absolute key to relieving and preventing recurrence of low back pain lies in strengthening the abdominal muscles. And by following the program laid out in this book, not only will you strengthen your abdominals, you will find that you look better and feel better as well.

In our physical therapy practice, we regularly treat back patients with the "Classic Eight," exercises that are detailed in Chapter 3. In addition to making rapid gains in abdominal firmness and strength, patients also improve their posture, transferring the benefits of exercise to practical everyday use as they walk, run, sit, and lift.

It continually amazes us to see our patients after they have been on this strengthening program. In a matter of a few short weeks, they look different, they stand more erect and relaxed, and, because they have firmed up their midsections, they move better, with more grace and power. This is quite apparent just watching them walk across a room.

64 MINUTES

This book details the same program we use with our patients at the Center for Sports and Osteopathic Medicine. Unlike other "no pain, all gain" books on the market, ours is a realistic, effective strategy designed for people who want to lose their midsection progressively and intelligently. When used consistently, our balanced approach to abdominal strengthening will firm and tone your weak abdominal muscles in just 16 minutes a day, four times a week, for a weekly total of just 64 minutes.

IT'S A "CINCH"

For most men, the part of the body that attracts most attention—good or bad—is the midsection. A toned middle not only adds structure to your silhouette, it can affect everything from the way you carry yourself to the confidence you exude.

Fortunately, the abdominal muscles are among the easiest to strengthen when you exercise them properly. In a matter of days you will feel the difference, usually marked by the ability to cinch up your belt one extra notch.

To go beyond that one notch, however, is going to take something else, and that something else is discipline—discipline to continue to do the stomach exercises on a regular basis, discipline to increase the exercise difficulty once they begin to feel too "comfortable," discipline to push yourself to the point of muscle fatigue, discipline to push yourself away from the table when you are feeling satisfied rather than stuffed.

Accordingly, the exercises in this book are flexibly designed to increase in difficulty so you can push yourself along as quickly as you are able. For instance, while the exercises remain the same, you can instantly move from beginner to intermediate to advanced levels just by changing your arm or leg position within the exercise. The philosophy behind this is that it is more rewarding to increase the efficiency of the exercises (all the while protecting the back) rather than expanding the time it takes to do them.

There are certain things that can't be changed in your body. Your height, the narrowness of your shoulders, the width of your hips are all predetermined at birth. However, as you will see, the size of your stomach is something you have a great deal of control over, and reducing its girth is a very realistic goal to shoot for. By following our abdominal strengthening program several times a week, you can progressively strengthen the abdominal muscles and pare away the fat that covers them.

MEN AND WOMEN: TALE OF THE FRUIT

It's hardly news that gender is the dominant factor in determining body type—with the "ideal" physique for women being the hourglass, and for men, the ramrod. It is also no surprise that men and women tend to add excess weight in different areas, men to their middle, women to their hips. Nutritionists and weight-control experts refer to these body types as apple-shaped for men and pear-shaped for women.

When it comes to flattening your stomach, this is both good and bad news for both men and women. The exercises in this book are specifically designed to be performed by either sex. But women should be aware that they may not be able to achieve the exact level of abdominal tone that they desire. In many cases, this limitation is due not to lack of trying, but to a matter of genetics. The "good news" for women is that while the stomach may be harder to tighten, there is less need to do so since this is not where the fat settles. (The hips and thighs, of course, are another story.) Conversely, men are more likely to see immediate, dramatic results, but they are also much more likely to need them.

The one obvious female exception to the above is in pregnant and postpartum women. Strong abdominals are a great help for pregnant women, whose muscles become stretched excessively during pregnancy. Super-strong abdominals act as a natural form-fitting girdle around the growing midsection to hold everything nicely in place, greatly reducing incidences of low back pain, and aiding in a smooth delivery.

After you give birth, your abdominal muscles remain extended and will sag noticeably. Once you have permission from your physician, begin the exercises at the beginner level for each exercise. Increase the repetitions and progress to higher levels as your strength and muscle endurance returns.

Don't be disappointed if you have trouble with the beginning level, or if you find that you can't finish the sets. As a new mother you will tire more easily. Don't give up. It will take time to get back to your prepregnancy figure and weight, but these exercises will certainly hasten the process.

THE ABDOMINALS: A QUICK PRIMER

Starting with getting out of bed in the morning, the abdominal muscles play a crucial role in how you move throughout the day. Bend. Twist. Turn. Sit down. Stand up. Lift your legs. Walk. With well-developed abdominals these movements are instinctive and come without effort.

The abdominal muscles encompass an area of the body starting at the ribs, down to slightly below the navel. They consist of four layers of overlapping fibers that crisscross the lower ribs, pelvis, and abdominal cavity diagonally, horizontally, and vertically. Their primary function is to provide movement to the trunk, as well as to keep the internal organs in place and to support the lower back.

The abdominal muscle group consists of four sinewy muscles: the *rectus abdominis,* the *external* and *internal obliques,* and the *transversus abdominis.*

The *rectus abdominis* is a long, flat muscle that extends along the whole length of the front of the torso, with horizontal tendons fanning out to the right and left. This is the prized muscle that receives all the attention from body builders, whose exercise routines make this muscle appear rippled.

The rectus abdominis inserts into the sternum, attaches to the fifth, sixth, and seventh ribs, and connects at the pubic bone just above the genitals. The *linea alba,* a half-inch-long tendon, separates the right and left halves of this muscle. This muscle helps you to lie down, sit, and get up. It does this by flexing the trunk, drawing the breastbone

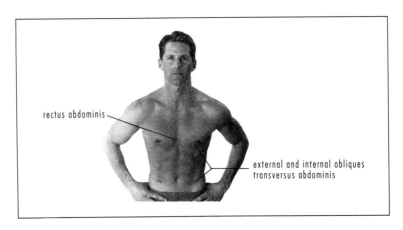

rectus abdominis

external and internal obliques
transversus abdominis

toward the pubic bone, and vice versa. The exercises outlined in this book will develop both the upper and lower portions of this muscle.

The oblique muscles define the waistline. The *external obliques* are the largest and most superficial of the abs. They run along the front and both sides of the abdomen from the lower eight ribs and insert into the crest of the pelvis. These muscles act to flex, side bend, and rotate the spine. The muscles come inward and meet the horizontal tendons of the rectus abdominis almost like a pair of hands, fingers apart, holding in the flanks. By performing the various oblique-strengthening exercises in this book, men will be able to make inroads on their "love handles," the fatty area just above the hips that is often difficult to remove.

The *internal oblique* muscles lie under the external obliques and mimic their function. The muscle rises from the crest of the pelvis and inserts into the lower four ribs.

The *transversus abdominis* lies under the internal oblique and runs the length of the abdomen, connecting from the lower six ribs to the pubic bone, which is located just above the genitals. This muscle helps with forced expiration of breath.

MORE THAN JUST A PRETTY GUT

In addition to the obvious cosmetic benefits of a flat stomach and a tight waist, there are a number of significant health benefits as well.

Your Life: Researchers have found that potbellies contribute to higher cholesterol levels, increase the risk of coronary artery disease, and can lead to adult onset diabetes. Research has shown this is linked to the fact that the more fat deposited in the abdominal region, the greater the chance that it will eventually work its way into the bloodstream. Health experts now estimate that for every inch that your waistline exceeds the size of your chest, you can deduct two years from your life expectancy.

Your Posture: Posture will be covered more fully in Chapter 5, but it is worth mentioning here that a strong stomach has both a physical *and* a psychological effect on posture. Strong abdominal muscles are crucial to holding the spine in proper alignment. Moreover, once you have gone to the effort of toning your stomach, you will not want to "ruin" the effect of your new straight-arrow physique by slouching. Once you become more aware of posture—how you look walking down the street—it will provide further motivation to keep the stomach tight and tucked in.

Your Back: As we have mentioned, underdeveloped abdominal muscles are one of the major causes of low back discomfort, weakness, stiffness, and pain. With an excess of fat tugging a weakened abdominal area forward, this extra weight throws the muscles supporting the spine out of whack. Eventually, this may lead to muscle spasm with back pain a direct result.

Your Performance: In addition to enhancing overall appearance with improved muscle tone, stronger abs will provide the strength and endurance needed to make improvements in athletic technique and overall sports performance.

AEROBICS AND DIET

It would be irresponsible for us to imply that maximum results can be attained simply by performing the exercises in Chapter 3. A perfectly toned midsection depends on a certain amount of aerobic exercise and nutritional considerations. Aerobic exercise, such as walking, running, swimming, and in-line skating, should be performed at least 20 minutes at a stretch, several times a week. We will review some aerobic strategies in more detail in Chapter 4.

As to nutrition, you do not have to go on a "diet" in order to lower your daily intake of calories from fats. Indeed, several fairly simple changes in your eating habits can lower fat intake dramatically. Chapter 7 provides some basic guidelines and commonsense eating tips.

Developing a flat, muscular stomach takes time, but even after your first workout your abdominal muscles will begin to feel different as they are called upon repeatedly to raise and lower your torso.

With each succeeding workout, you will feel and then start to see the difference as the various abdominal muscles become stronger and more defined. Of course, changing your body takes time, but no matter what shape you're in at the start of the program, within twelve weeks you will see major results.

HOW DO YOU MEASURE UP?

One of the factors related to high cholesterol and high blood pressure readings is the amount of fat you have stored in the abdominal area. A quick way to find out how much you have is to determine your waist-to-hip ratio. If your waist girth is greater than your hips, then you have too much fat and need to lose it. Our program will help you do this safely and efficiently.

To compute your waist-to-hip ratio and determine your current health risk:
- Without clothing, measure around your waist at navel level to the nearest quarter inch.
- Measure around your hips at the buttocks to the nearest quarter inch. Take several readings at various levels. Use the largest one for the equation.
- Divide the waist number by the hip number.
- Your hips should be larger than your waist. For women, the waist-to-hip ratio should be less than 0.80, for males less than 0.90.

2

Getting Started

Abdominal exercise has come a long way from the classic sit-up, which not only produced a lot of wasted motion but was more likely to cause back pain than to prevent it.

Your abdominal program will consist of a strengthening routine based on the techniques we use with patients at the Center for Sports and Osteopathic Medicine in New York City. We call these abdominal exercises the Classic Eight. For best results we recommend that the entire program be performed at least four times a week. The exercises include:

Abdominal crunch
Crossed leg oblique
Leg drop oblique
Advanced leg drop oblique

Bicycle progression
Forward leg drop progression
Reverse sit-up
Pop-up

FOLLOW THE EXERCISE SEQUENCE

These abdominal exercises are designed to be followed in sequence because they increase in difficulty as you move from one to the next. However, once you progress to the advanced level, your abs will be sufficiently strengthened to perform the more difficult exercises out of sequence if you choose.

ONLY 16 MINUTES FROM YOUR BUSY SCHEDULE

Each exercise session will last no longer than 16 minutes. You will perform the eight specific abdominal exercises, each consisting of three sets of fifteen repetitions. During this time, you will be strengthening *only* your abdominal muscles, working them until you think that you can't perform another repetition.

Granted, 16 minutes is a lot of time to spend on just one body part, but in order to achieve the most gains, you have to work the abdominal muscle fibers beyond your typical everyday demands.

YOUR TRAINING LEVEL

Finding the specific exercise level to suit your abilities is very simple. The following will help you to choose correctly.

BEGINNER LEVEL

If you have never exercised, if you are in poor physical condition, or if you are overweight, start at this level and perform 3 sets of 5 repetitions of each exercise. All exercises should be performed with the arms kept at the sides. Once you become stronger and find that this becomes too easy, that the abs don't fatigue, and the abdominal contractions can be held without difficulty, perform 3 sets of 10 repetitions. When this eventually becomes too easy, move to 3 sets

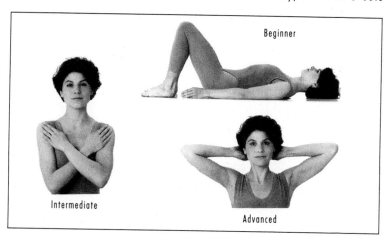

Beginner

Intermediate

Advanced

of 15. It's time to go to the intermediate level when you are no longer significantly challenged.

INTERMEDIATE LEVEL

If you have graduated from the beginner level, or if you already exercise with some regularity and find the beginner level too easy but the advanced level too strenuous, then the intermediate level is for you.

Start at this level with 3 sets of 10 repetitions. The arms should be crossed over the chest for most of the exercises and the intermediate leg positions should be used. Once you can make it through the workout and find that the abs don't fatigue, and the contractions can be held without difficulty, perform 3 sets of 15 reps. When you reach the point where this no longer taxes your muscles, you are ready to move to the advanced level.

ADVANCED LEVEL

If you have graduated from the intermediates, or if you are already in great physical shape with a strong midsection, start at this level. Perform 3 sets of 10 reps of the exercises. The hands should be kept behind the head during most of the exercises. Don't interlace your fingers. Keep your elbows flared straight out from your torso and use advanced leg positions when applicable. Perform 3 sets of 15 reps when the 10-rep sets no longer tax your abdominals sufficiently.

THE IMPORTANCE OF PROPER TECHNIQUE

Follow the instructions for each exercise very carefully. To get maximum waistline benefit you must perform each exercise according to the instructions, using proper technique. Remember, too, you get better results the more *slowly* you perform each contraction.

For a quick reminder, refer to the exercise descriptions in the book as you go along so you can keep the exercises flowing from one to the next without losing your momentum. You will find after you have completed the workout several times that you will be able to remember the exercise positions and the sequence.

BREATHING

Proper breathing technique plays a very important role in this program. During each repetition of an exercise, inhale just before you start the exertion phase. Exhale slowly as you go through the exertion. Never hold your breath between repetitions of an exercise. This could make you feel light-headed or faint.

THE ABDOMINAL CONTRACTION

As you perform the exercises in Chapter 3 it is important to focus on the abdominal muscles. Not only is the abdominal contraction an isometric exercise unto itself, it dramatically improves the efficiency of the abdominal exercise thereby hastening noticeable results in the streamlining of your midsection.

Begin by inhaling deeply through your nose. As you exhale the natural tendency is to let your abdominal muscles go limp. You must consciously fight this tendency by tensing the abdominal muscles. Anatomically the idea is to lower the ribs down toward the belly button while simultaneously lifting the pubic (groin) bone up toward the belly button. You should also maintain a slight arch in your back. The abdominal contraction is not as complicated as it may sound. In order to feel the results you are looking for, cough deeply a couple of times; the tightening of the abdominal muscles just as you cough approxi-

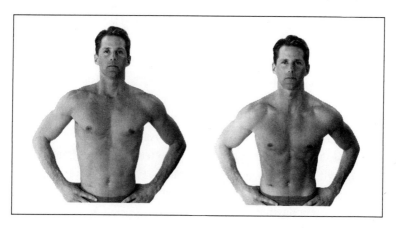

mates the sensation you are looking for. You should also feel the isometric pressure against the rib cage and the groin area from this contraction.

For every exercise the breathing rhythm is this: inhale deeply as your body is at rest, then exhale and contract simultaneously as you lean into the exercise.

Once this contraction is learned, it should be utilized not just for the exercises, but during sitting, standing, and walking throughout the day. As a result, you will be strengthening your abdominals every time you consciously make an effort to contract them.

REPS AND SETS

A repetition or "rep" is the number of times that you perform the same exercise from beginning to end of a set. We have found that beginners performing 10 repetitions of each exercise for 3 sets—a set is a number of reps performed without stopping—is best for building stronger, defined abdominals. As you get stronger, increase reps to 15 per exercise.

REST BETWEEN SETS

You should rest for at least 30 seconds between each set to allow your working muscles time to recuperate after being pushed to the max. If you skip the rest period or cut it short, you may not have sufficient strength to make it through the next set. The end result may be a shortened workout and fewer gains for your efforts.

OVERCOMING DELAYED ONSET MUSCLE SORENESS

Focusing all the exercises on just the abdominal muscles for 16-minute bouts will start bringing results the first day. More visible effects in the midsection will be evident within a short while.

After your first workout your abdominal muscles are going to feel different. In subsequent workouts you will probably feel a burning sensation in this area. A few hours later, the next day, or even two days later, the midsection may still ache. This is called delayed onset muscle soreness and it's a normal reaction to strenuous exercise. Within a few days this soreness should disappear.

Take pleasure in this feeling. It serves as a reminder that you are really getting results from the workout, and that you are pushing your muscles to grow. Despite abdominal muscle soreness, you can still continue with the program. Although it seems contradictory, the more you pump blood through the abdominal area with further exercise, the better you will feel.

To minimize muscle soreness, start at the beginner level with each exercise. Once the abdominals have become accustomed to the exercises and you can perform the entire routine to completion, increase your repetitions, or move on to the next level.

If the soreness doesn't lessen or disappear after a few days, or if you feel any unusually sharp pain in the abdomen as you exercise, stop the exercise and consult your physician.

WHEN IS THE BEST TIME TO EXERCISE?

Many people find that exercising right after they get out of bed in the morning is the best time to exercise. By immediately getting exercise out of the way, you don't have the specter of ''I've got to do my exercises!'' hanging over your head throughout the day.

We are not doctrinaire when it comes to exercise time. The best time for you is whenever you can fit it into your schedule. If you happen to be a morning person and full of pep, then work out in the morning. However, if you feel too stiff first thing out of bed, wait until you have been up for a while and are more flexible. If you have time during your lunch break or when you come home from work, try to exercise then. A big plus for P.M. workouts is they can help you to blow off the accumulated tension and stress of the day. Work out shortly before dinner and you may find that your appetite is reduced.

A final note on when to exercise: try to establish a schedule so that you work out at approximately the same time every day. This helps to "ritualize" the workout. Of course, if you can't do your routine at that time, commit yourself immediately to another time that same day. The most important thing is not *when* you exercise, but that you *do* exercise.

Pick the time that best meets your needs. And when you find you are finally ready, put on some music, turn on your answering machine, and go for it.

WHAT CLOTHES SHOULD BE WORN?

The emphasis here is on total comfort. This may mean a T-shirt and gym shorts, a leotard, a running suit, even pajamas. The important thing is to wear whatever you want as long as total range of motion of the arms and legs is not restricted.

SHOES OR NO SHOES?

Go shoeless if you are just beginning the program and don't want any added resistance as you perform the exercises. For a tougher workout, wearing athletic shoes while you perform the exercises will add more resistance to the workout and make the exercises even more challenging. Moving your leg up and down with a half-pound shoe on it may not seem like a difficult task initially, but as the workout progresses, that same shoe will feel much heavier to your fatiguing muscles when you perform the forward leg drop, the bicycle, and the pop-up.

Additional resistance can also be added by wearing ankle weights on all leg-lift exercises. These strap-on weights are available in sporting goods stores in various weight denominations. If you are going to use the weights, make sure that they're not so heavy that they keep you from completing your three sets of each exercise.

3

The Classic Eight Abdominal Exercises

Since you will probably perform the Classic Eight program by yourself, the success of this strengthening regimen depends totally on you. Learn to listen to your body, noting how you feel during and after a workout. Pay attention to your overall condition, the signs of early fatigue, or how sore your abdominals become. Remember too, as we discussed in Chapter 2, that the ache you may feel in your muscles is a temporary condition that will be relieved by more exercise, and should completely disappear in a matter of days.

Strengthening for the Upper Abdominals: 1. The Abdominal Crunch

F O R M
- Lie on your back, knees bent, feet resting on the exercise mat.
- Choose an arm position suitable for your current conditioning (see page 12).

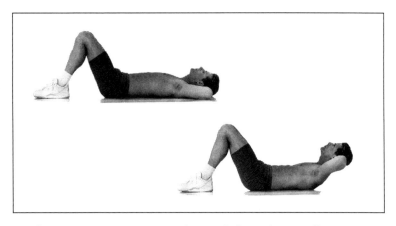

- Make sure your nose is pointed toward the ceiling at all times.

EXECUTION
- Inhale deeply.
- Upon exhalation, contract your abdominals and allow them simultaneously to lift your head and shoulders off the exercise mat.
- Rise up slowly until your shoulder blades are just clear of the mat.
- Slowly, in a controlled fashion, allow your shoulders and head to return to the mat.
- Repeat the sequence until you have finished your set.

OPTION: ABDOMINAL CRUNCH USING A BENCH

Another option for beginner-level exercisers is to use a chair, bench, or couch. For better abdominal muscle control, place your lower legs on a bench, across the seat of a low chair, or on a couch. Perform the crunch exercise as described above.

Progress through the three arm positions (see page 12). Once you can eventually complete the crunch sets in the advanced arm position, perform the exercise without the chair.

EXERCISE POINTERS
- Do not hook your legs under a chair or couch, or allow someone to hold your feet on the floor. This lets the hip flexor muscles take

over for the abdominals and lessens the effectiveness of the crunch.

- Be sure to move your neck and head together as one unit. Don't jerk your head upward as you raise your shoulders up off the mat; this may strain your neck.
- Don't arch your back. This may compress your lower vertebrae and lead to tenderness in the area.
- As you strengthen at each level, come up slightly higher and increase the force of the abdominal contraction.
- The slower and more controlled you return to the rest position, the more effective the movement and the more dramatic the end results will be.

Strengthening for the Oblique Abdominals: 2. The Crossed Leg Oblique

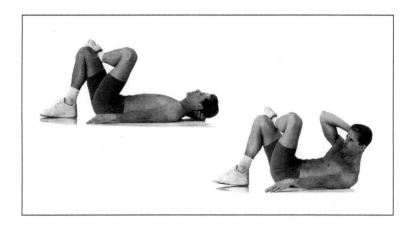

FORM

- Lie on your back with the right knee bent and right foot flat on the mat.

- Cross the left leg over the right, with the ankle resting on the thigh of the right leg.
- Choose an arm position suitable for your current conditioning.

E X E C U T I O N
- Inhale deeply.
- Upon exhalation, contract the abdominals and allow them to slowly lift the head and shoulder diagonally up toward the elevated left knee. Go high enough to clear the shoulder blade from the mat.
- Slowly and in a controlled manner, return to the starting position.
- Repeat the sequence until you have finished your set.
- On alternate sets, perform by crossing your opposite leg.

E X E R C I S E P O I N T E R S
- The arm on the side of the elevated knee should be extended out to the side and resting on the mat.
- Be sure to move your neck and head together as one unit. Don't jerk your head upward as you raise your shoulders up off the mat; this may strain your neck.
- Don't arch your back. This may compress your vertebrae and lead to tenderness in the area.
- As you strengthen at each level, come up slightly higher with the shoulders and increase the force of the abdominal contraction.
- The slower and more controlled you return to the rest position, the more effective the movement and the more dramatic the abdominal strengthening will be.

3. Leg Drop Oblique

F O R M
- Lie on your back with knees bent and feet flat on the mat in line with the buttocks.
- Choose an arm position suitable for your current conditioning (see page 12).

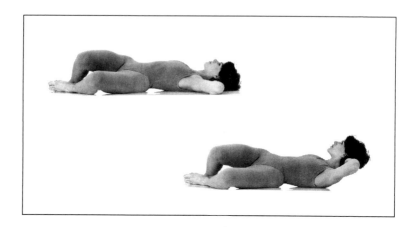

- Keep your nose pointed directly at the ceiling throughout the exercise.
- Keeping feet in line with buttocks, slowly drop one leg outward onto the mat and follow with the opposite leg so that it now rests on top.
- Don't "curl" your upper torso. Keep lengthened between the ribs and pelvis on the side opposite the leg drop.

EXECUTION

- Inhale deeply.
- Upon exhalation, contract abdominals and allow them slowly to lift head and shoulders off the mat.
- Slowly and in a controlled manner, return to the start.
- Repeat the sequence until you have finished your set.
- On alternate sets, perform by dropping your legs on the other side of your body.

EXERCISE POINTERS

- Be sure to move your neck and head together as one unit. Don't jerk your head upward as you raise your shoulders up off the mat; this may strain your neck.
- Don't arch your back. This may compress your vertebrae and lead to tenderness in the area.

- As you strengthen at each level, come up slightly higher and increase the force of the abdominal contraction.
- The slower and more controlled you return to the start position, the more effective the movement and the more dramatic the end results will be.

4. Advanced Leg Drop Oblique

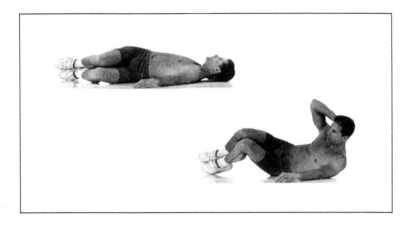

FORM
- Lie on your back with knees bent and feet flat on the mat.
- Use an arm position suitable for your current conditioning (see page 12).
- Keeping your feet in line with your buttocks, slowly drop one leg outward onto the floor or mat and follow with the opposite leg until both legs are as close to the mat as possible.
- Keep lengthened between ribs and pelvis on the side opposite leg drop.

EXECUTION
- Inhale deeply.
- Upon exhalation, contract abdominals and allow them slowly to lift head and shoulders and move diagonally toward dropped knees.

- Simultaneously rotate both knees toward the opposite side.
- Slowly and in a controlled fashion, allow your shoulders and legs to return to the mat.
- Repeat the sequence until you have finished your set.
- On alternate sets, perform by dropping your legs on the other side of your body.

EXERCISE POINTERS

- Use three arm positions as needed, but make sure that the arm on the side of the knee drop is extended out to the side and resting on the mat.
- Don't jerk your head upward; this will strain your neck. Be sure to move your neck and head together as one unit.
- Don't arch your back. This may compress your vertebrae and lead to tenderness in the area.
- This is a difficult exercise. However, as you strengthen at each level, come up slightly higher and increase the force of the abdominal contraction.
- The slower and more controlled you return to the rest position, the more effective the movement and the more dramatic the end results will be.

Strengthening for the Lower Abdominals: 5. The Bicycle Progression

FORM

- Lie on your back with knees bent and feet flat on the mat.
- Slowly lift both knees toward the chest, one at a time.

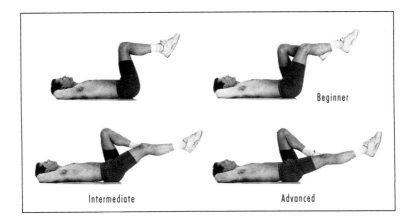

Beginner

Intermediate   Advanced

EXECUTION

There are three progressions in the bicycle exercise. Advance to the next level only when the contraction can be held without the arms supporting the low back, the low back doesn't arch, and when all three sets seem too easy.

• Inhale deeply.
• Slowly exhale and contract the abdominals.

Beginner Progression
• Bring knees toward the chest (90/90 degrees).

Intermediate Progression
• Legs move to mid range.

Advanced Progression
• Legs are almost parallel to the floor, always maintaining a slight knee bend, back not arching.

• While maintaining the abdominal contraction and continuing to breathe normally, slowly move legs slightly forward and then back, one at a time, in a bicycle pedaling motion.
• Keep knees bent and hips extended forward.
• A repetition is counted after both legs have been extended.
• Repeat the sequence until you have finished the set.

EXERCISE POINTERS

- Maintain a strong contraction so the low back is not allowed to arch.
- Maintain a short range of motion in the legs.
- Use a pillow under your head to keep from straining the neck muscles.
- If necessary, support the low back with your hands. However, if a proper abdominal contraction is held, this should not be required.
- As you strengthen your abdominals over time, work the legs even more slowly for more dramatic abdominal results.

6. Forward Leg Drop Progression

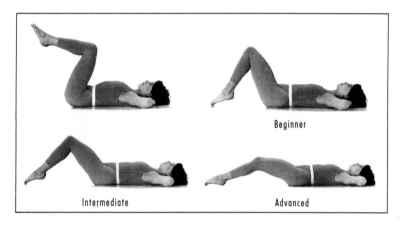

Beginner

Intermediate   Advanced

FORM

- Lie on your back with knees bent and feet flat on the mat.
- Keep your arms at your sides or behind your head.

EXECUTION

There are three progressions in the forward leg drop. Advance to the next level when the abdominal contraction seems too easy and you can perform this exercise without arching your back.

- Draw both knees up toward the chest one at a time.

- Inhale deeply.
- Upon exhalation, contract the abdominals strongly.

Beginner Level
- While maintaining the contraction and continuing normal breathing, keep both legs close together and slowly lower the legs to the mat while keeping the knees bent.
- Move legs forward until the toes gently touch the floor.

Intermediate Level
- Drop your toes to the mat approximately two feet out from your buttocks.

Advanced Level
- Keep a slight bend in your knee.
- Drop your *heels* as far out from your buttocks as you can comfortably go without arching your back.

- As soon as the toes touch, return the legs slowly toward the chest.
- Repeat the sequence until you have finished the set.
- After each set, return the feet to the floor with knees bent.

EXERCISE POINTERS
- Maintain a strong contraction so the low back is not allowed to arch.
- Use a pillow under your head to keep from straining the neck muscles.
- If necessary, support the low back with your hands. However, if a proper abdominal contraction is held, this should not be required.
- As you strengthen the abdominals over time, work the legs even more slowly for more dramatic abdominal results.
- After each set, return the feet to the floor one at a time while keeping the knees bent.

7. Reverse Sit-Up

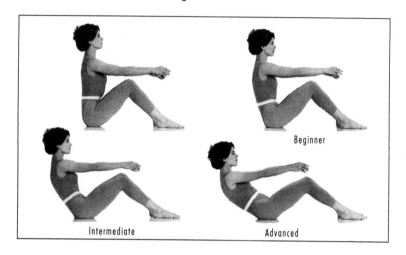

Beginner

Intermediate

Advanced

FORM

- Sit on the mat with knees bent and feet flat on the mat.
- Choose an arm position suitable for your current conditioning (see page 12).

EXECUTION

- Inhale deeply.

Beginner Level

- Upon exhalation, and with strong abdominal control, very slowly allow the abdominals to lower your back 30 degrees toward the mat.

Intermediate Level

- Lower your back 60 degrees toward the mat.

Advanced Level

- Lower your back approximately 12 inches from the mat.
- Return to starting position without using your hands to push off the mat. If you start to fatigue, use your hands.
- Repeat the sequence until you have finished your set.

EXERCISE POINTERS

- Maintain a strong abdominal contraction.
- Keep your head relaxed and in line with your spine.
- Don't bring your chin toward your chest. Keep your eyes focused forward.
- Don't twist from side to side or let your back arch as you come back up. When you arch your back this reduces the forces on the abdominals and puts them on the hip flexors and low back.
- As you strengthen your abdominals over time, descend even more slowly for more dramatic abdominal results.

8. Pop-Up

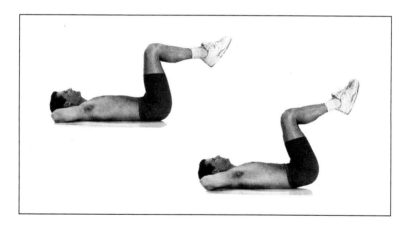

FORM

- Lie on the mat with knees bent and feet flat on the mat.
- Bring knees up toward the chest, one at a time to a 90 degree/ 90 degree position, knees facing ceiling.

EXECUTION

- Inhale deeply.

- Upon exhalation, contract abdominals and lift buttocks *straight up* off the mat solely by contracting the lower abdominals.
- After you have gone up as far as you can, slowly and in a controlled fashion return to the starting position.
- Repeat the sequence until you have finished the set.

EXERCISE POINTERS

- This is the most difficult exercise in the Classic Eight. Pretend that your legs are going straight up the wall, propelled by your abdominal muscles.
- Knees should remain facing the ceiling throughout the exercise.
- Do not allow legs or buttocks to roll toward the chest.
- Do not push up with your hands.
- Use a pillow under your head to avoid straining the neck muscles.

WORKOUT POINTERS

SLOW AND STEADY

You will achieve maximum results when you perform each repetition slowly and in complete control.

When you "cheat" on an exercise by using your arms to bounce up, or by rocking back quickly off your back or side, you will lessen the effectiveness of the exercise. If you begin to fatigue and can't complete a set without "cheating," then cut back on the number of reps, or switch to a different training level.

DON'T HOLD YOUR BREATH

Inhale completely as you begin each exercise and exhale as you perform the motion. Do not hold your breath or you may feel dizzy or light-headed.

DON'T PUSH THROUGH PAIN

These are demanding exercises and will produce startling results. However, if you become extremely tired during an exercise session, slow down, or stop and take a break. If you experience abnormal pain or soreness at any point, stop the exercise.

4

The Program

As you probably know already from past experience, the hard part of exercise is sticking with a program. As mentioned earlier, we generally believe that there is no best time to perform these exercises. Obviously, it is not so important *when* you do these exercises but that you *do* them. However, performing these exercises first thing in the morning leaves you without the specter of performing them hanging over your head all day and prevents you from rationalizing skipping a session as the day wears on.

What you will find is that beyond the first several filled-with-commitment sessions the initial sessions will require a great deal of discipline. But as with most other things, as the habit begins to take hold you will find these sessions will become more and more automatic. After several weeks, once you begin to see results, you will find that the process becomes reversed: if you don't do the exercises it will seem that your day is incomplete.

GENERAL PROGRAM GUIDELINES

The exercise program recommended here assumes three distinct levels of fitness and progresses from one to the next as your abdominal muscles get stronger. If you are already in pretty good or very good shape you may want to begin at the intermediate or advanced level, but don't try to do too much too soon. This will only discourage you, perhaps to the point of skipping sessions altogether.

The three levels of this program are briefly described below.

Beginning level. Incorporates four exercises—crunch, crossed leg oblique, bicycle progressions, and reverse sit-ups (Program exercises 1–4)—which gradually increase in repetitions. If you are so inclined, exercises at this level can be done on a daily basis.

Exercising at these low-intensity levels allows the body to adapt safely, progressively, and comfortably to the stresses and demands of the different exercises. You can stay with this entry level as long as you like, changing the order of exercises to fit your mood. As your conditioning increases over the weeks, you can move to the more demanding intermediate level.

Intermediate level. This level uses a higher level of intensity and more advanced arm and leg positions for the first four exercises—crunch, crossed leg oblique, bicycle progressions, and reverse sit-ups—to bring about greater resistance, and adds two additional exercises, the leg drop oblique and forward leg drop (Program exercises 5–6). Start the program at week 3 on the chart (2 sets of 5 reps in the number 2 arm and leg positions) or week 5 for the more advanced exercises within this level and follow it through to the end. You may stay with this level as long as you like, but for greater challenge, move to the advanced level.

Advanced level. If you have been exercising regularly and already have strong abdominals, begin the program at week 7 with the first four exercises—crunch, crossed leg oblique, bike progressions, and reverse sit-ups (2 sets of 5 reps with the advanced arm and leg positions) and the leg drop oblique and forward leg drop (2 sets of 10–15 reps). For a greater challenge, move on to week 11 where the final two (and most difficult) exercises are added—advanced leg drop oblique and pop-up (Program exercises 7–8).

THE TWELVE WEEKS

The following sample chart is set up in three 4-week increments, each progressing but generally reflecting a beginning, intermediate, and advanced level of fitness.

MONTH 1

B E G I N N E R   L E V E L
Exercises   Crunch, crossed leg oblique, bicycle progression, reverse sit-up (exercises 1–4)

Beginner Positions
• Arms: at sides for all exercises
• Legs: knees toward chest for bicycle, first position for reverse sit-up (no. 1 arm and leg positions)

W E E K   1

Day 1	2 sets of 5 reps using the no. 1 arm and leg positions
Day 2	Same
Day 3	Rest
Day 4	2 sets of 5–10 reps using no. 1 positions
Day 5	Rest
Day 6	Same
Day 7	Rest

W E E K   2

Day 8	2 sets of 10 reps using no. 1 positions
Day 9	Same
Day 10	Rest
Day 11	Same
Day 12	Rest
Day 13	2 sets of 10–15 reps using no. 1 positions
Day 14	Rest

Intermediate Positions
- Arms: across chest
- Legs: mid-position; second position for reverse sit-up (no. 2 arm and leg positions)

BEGINNER/INTERMEDIATE LEVEL

WEEK 3

Day 15	2 sets of 5–10 reps using no. 1 positions, or 2 sets of 5 reps using no. 2 positions
Day 16	Same
Day 17	Rest
Day 18	2 sets of 15 reps using no. 1 positions, or 2 sets of 5 reps using no. 2 positions
Day 19	Rest
Day 20	Same
Day 21	Rest

WEEK 4

Day 22	2 sets of 15 reps using no. 1 positions, or 2 sets of 5–10 reps using no. 2 positions
Day 23	2 sets of 15–20 reps using no. 1 positions, or 2 sets of 5–10 reps using no. 2 positions
Day 24	Rest
Day 25	Same
Day 26	Rest
Day 27	Same
Day 28	Rest

MONTH 2

INTERMEDIATE LEVEL

Exercises Crunch, crossed leg oblique, bicycle progression, reverse sit-up (exercises 1–4); forward leg drop, leg drop oblique (exercises 5–6)

WEEK 5

Day 1	Exercises 1–4: 2 sets of 20 reps using no. 1 positions or 2 sets of 10 reps using no. 2 positions Exercises 5–6: 2 sets of 5 reps using no. 1 positions
Day 2	Same
Day 3	Rest
Day 4	Same
Day 5	Rest
Day 6	Same
Day 7	Rest

WEEK 6

Day 8	Exercises 1–4: Same, or 2 sets of 10–15 reps using no. 2 positions Exercises 5–6: 2 sets of 5–10 reps using no. 1 positions
Day 9	Same
Day 10	Rest
Day 11	Same, except exercises 5–6: 2 sets of 10 reps using no. 1 positions
Day 12	Rest
Day 13	Same
Day 14	Rest

Advanced Positions
• Arms: behind head
• Legs: close to floor; third position for reverse sit-up (no. 3 leg positions)

INTERMEDIATE/ADVANCED LEVEL

WEEK 7

Day 15	Exercise 1–4: 3 sets of 15 reps using no. 1 positions, or 2 sets of 15 reps using no. 2 positions, or 2 sets of 5 reps using no. 3 positions Exercises 5–6: 2 sets of 10–15 reps using no. 1 positions
Day 16	Same
Day 17	Rest

Day 18 Same
Day 19 Rest
Day 20 Same
Day 21 Rest

Once 3 sets of 15 reps can be performed without difficulty, the beginner positions can be eliminated.

Day 22 Exercises 1–4: 2 sets of 15–20 reps using no. 2 positions, or 2 sets of 5–10 reps using no. 3 positions
Exercises 5–6: 2 sets of 15 reps using no. 1 positions, or 2 sets of 5 reps using no. 2 positions

WEEK 8

Day 23 Same
Day 24 Rest
Day 25 Same
Day 26 Rest
Day 27 Same
Day 28 Rest

MONTH 3

WEEK 9

Day 1 Exercises 1–4: 2 sets of 20 reps using no. 2 positions, or 2 sets of 10–15 reps using no. 3 positions
Exercises 5–6: 2 sets of 15–20 reps using no. 1 positions, or 2 sets of 5–10 reps using no. 2 positions
Day 2 Same
Day 3 Rest
Day 4 Same
Day 5 Rest
Day 6 Same
Day 7 Rest

WEEK 10

Day 8 Exercises 1–4: 3 sets of 15 reps using no. 2 positions, or 2 sets of 15 reps using no. 3 positions

Exercises 5–6: 2 sets of 20 reps using no. 1 positions, or 2 sets of 10 reps using no. 2 positions

Day 9   Same
Day 10   Rest
Day 11   Same
Day 12   Rest
Day 13   Same
Day 14   Rest

Once 3 sets of 15 reps can be performed without difficulty, the intermediate positions can be eliminated.

ADVANCED LEVEL

Exercises   At this level you will gently start to incorporate the last two exercises into the program. These are the advanced leg drop oblique and the pop-up (exercises 7–8).

WEEK 11

Day 15   Exercises 1–4: 2 sets of 15–20 reps using no. 3 positions
              Exercises 5–6: 3 sets of 15 reps using no. 1 positions, or 2 sets of 10–15 reps using no. 2 positions, or 2 sets of 5 reps using no. 3 positions
              Exercises 7–8: 2 sets of 5 reps using no. 1 positions
Day 16   Same
Day 17   Rest
Day 18   Same
Day 19   Rest
Day 20   Same
Day 21   Rest

WEEK 12

Day 22   Exercises 1–4: 2 sets of 20 reps using no. 3 positions
              Exercises 5–6: 2 sets of 15 reps using no. 2 positions, or 2 sets of 5–10 reps using no. 3 positions
              Exercises 7–8: 2 sets of 5–10 reps using no. 1 positions
Day 23   Same
Day 24   Rest
Day 25   Same

Day 26 Rest
Day 27 Exercises 1–4: 3 sets of 15 reps using no. 3 positions
Exercises 5–6: 2 sets of 15–20 reps using no. 2 positions
or 2 sets of 10 reps using no. 3 positions
Exercises 7–8: 2 sets of 10 reps using no. 1 positions
Day 28 Rest

As you enter this phase of your program, the crossed leg oblique and leg drop oblique exercises may be eliminated. Remember to continue to work up to at least 3 sets of 15 of all your exercises.

Your advanced-level program will include:
Abdominal crunch
Advanced leg drop oblique
Bicycle progression
Forward leg drop
Reverse sit-up
Pop-up

INCORPORATING THE CLASSIC EIGHT INTO A NO-EQUIPMENT GENERAL CONDITIONING PROGRAM

While our abdominal program will strengthen your midsection, we recommend that this be incorporated into a general conditioning program that will not only help you firm up through aerobic exercise but will also improve general muscle tone and help prevent injury. The following sample exercise routine is a basic one that we often give to our patients.

GENERAL CONDITIONING LIST
Day 1 Abdominals (Classic Eight)
Aerobics (walk, run, bike, etc.), 20 minutes
Upper body workout (push-up), 5 minutes
Stretching, 5 minutes

Day 2	Abdominals
	Lower body workout (lunges, squats), 5 minutes
	Stretching, 5 minutes
Day 3	Aerobics, 20 minutes
	Upper body workout, 5 minutes
	Stretching, 5 minutes
Day 4	Abdominals
	Lower body workout, 5 minutes
	Stretching, 5 minutes
Day 5	Rest; however, stretching can be done on this day if so desired
Day 6	Abdominals
	Aerobics, 20 minutes
	Upper body workout, 5 minutes
	Stretching, 5 minutes
Day 7	Aerobics, 20 minutes
	Lower body workout, 5 minutes
	Stretching, 5 minutes

PROGRAM GUIDELINES

• The program provides for four weekly abdominal workouts along with a variety of aerobic suggestions and upper and lower body exercises. If you are pressed for time, focus only on the abdominals that particular day.

• Upper and lower body exercises are separated by a day to allow for full recovery.

• There is one rest day scheduled. Use this day to give your body a chance to recover fully from the stresses of the program. If you find yourself particularly tired, take extra time off.

As you can see, aerobic exercise is also included in this program. The mix of abdominal strength training with aerobic exercises such as walking, swimming, or bicycling helps promote fat loss and weight loss. Performing one or more of these activities for at least 20 minutes several times during the week is all that it takes to achieve sustained health benefits.

WARMING UP

A warm-up is recommended before beginning the aerobic exercises in order to increase body temperature and blood circulation as well as prepare the muscles for the upcoming demands. A warm-up helps prevent injury: cold muscles are stiff and liable to become damaged if you suddenly make vigorous demands of them.

Exercises such as jumping jacks, side bends, rope skipping, stationary bicycling, walking, or jogging are great for getting the blood circulating. Once the warm-up is completed, you should be perspiring lightly and ready to begin.

THE UPPER EXTREMITY EXERCISES

P U S H-U P
• Lie with your stomach on the floor, hands at your sides, palms facing downward, elbows in line with your legs.
• Keep your body rigid and push yourself upward until your arms straighten.
• Lower yourself until your chest touches the floor.
• Push upward and repeat.
• Beginner level: 1 set of 10 reps.
• Intermediate level: Start with 2 sets of 10 reps.
• Advanced level: 3 sets of 10 reps.

THE LOWER EXTREMITY EXERCISES

L U N G E
• Stand straight with feet shoulder-width apart.
• Step forward with your right leg and descend until the upper thigh is parallel to the floor.
• Return to the starting position.
• Complete the set and repeat with the left leg.
• Beginner level: Perform 1 set of 10 reps with each leg.
• Intermediate level: Perform 2 sets of 10 reps with each leg.
• Advanced level: 3 sets of 10.

WEIGHTLESS SQUATS

- Stand with feet shoulder-width apart.
- Cross your arms out in front of your chest.
- Slowly descend until your thighs are parallel to the floor.
- Pause momentarily.
- Forcefully push back up to the start position without twisting or turning the knees.
- Beginner level: 1 set of 10 reps.
- Intermediate level: 1 set of 15 reps.
- Advanced level: 2 sets of 15–20 reps.

5

Posture

When the subject of posture came up during our training, the professor looked around the classroom and announced that of the thirty-five physical therapy students sitting there, only one of us was sitting in a way that remotely resembled good posture.

Good posture is something that has to be worked on every day until it becomes a habit. But once you have attained it you will not only have lessened your risk of back pain, you will breathe easier and look better.

Most of us do not even know what good posture "feels" like. So in brief:

Standing: Come to military "attention." Now, while holding that position, relax. Your posture should not be as exaggerated as a drill sergeant's, but it will have some basic similarities: shoulders back, chest out, eyes focused forward, chin parallel to the floor, pelvis upright, feet firmly on the floor. You should also allow for the slight natural curvatures of your spine.

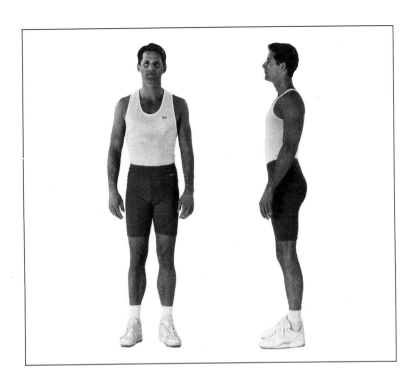

Walking: Walking is nothing more than standing posture in motion, with the only change coming from the arms, which gently swing in opposition to your legs as you walk.

WALKING EXERCISE

Stand a few inches from a wall with your feet 6–8 inches apart. Contract your abdominal muscles but not your buttocks. While breathing normally, gently place your shoulder blades against the wall. With the shoulders on the wall, your neck and head should automatically fall into good postural alignment.

Make sure your chin is parallel to the floor and that your focus is level, your earlobes are directly over your shoulders, your shoulders are over your hips, and your hips are directly over your knees. Knees should be relaxed, directly over the instep of your feet.

Hold this position for 30 seconds. Walk away from the wall and try to hold this posture for as long as possible. Repeat the exercise.

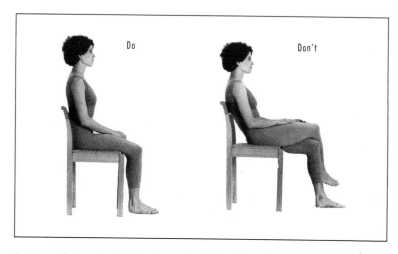

Do   Don't

Sitting: The seat of the chair should be high enough so your thighs rest horizontally on the seat. Feet should be flat on the floor with your knees directly over your feet. Earlobes should be over your shoulders. Make sure your chin is parallel to the floor and your focus is level. Keep the abdominal muscles gently contracted to form a natural girdle around the entire midsection. With proper sitting posture you should be able to "feel" your two "seat bones" (ischial tuberosities).

POSTURE KEYS

We find that in teaching our patients good posture it is helpful to have them focus on only one visual image or "key" that opens the door to proper overall alignment. Here are some of the images that we know have worked for our patients:

- Imagine that your neck and spine are forming a straight line perpendicular to the ground.
- As you move, pretend you are sandwiched between two panes of glass with no room for any bulges from your buttocks, abdomen, or slumping shoulders.
- Pretend that your head is filled with helium and that it floats upward, holding your neck and spine in alignment.
- Lift your chest as if walking proudly.

POOR POSTURE SIGNALS

Check yourself from time to time throughout the day for the following postural flaws.

Abdomen: Does your abdomen stick out in front? Perform the abdominal contraction (page 14) to pull it back.

Buttocks: Do they project out too far in the rear? Pull your shoulders back, contract your abdominal muscles, and straighten your torso.

Shoulders: Are they rounded and slumped forward? Gently pull your shoulders back and make sure your focus is level, chin parallel to the floor.

Chest: Does it appear sunken and collapsed? Pull your shoulders back and perform the abdominal contraction.

Neck: Does it feel "short" and tight? Make sure your focus is level and your chin parallel to the floor. This will cause the back of the neck to feel "long."

Head: Does your head tilt forward or to the side? Make sure your chin is parallel to the floor, your focus level, and your earlobes directly over your shoulders.

6

The Five-Minute Stretch

It is generally believed that it is good to perform a stretching routine prior to exercise or strenuous athletic activity. Researchers have found, however, that it is more useful and injury-preventative to perform some exercise that gets your blood flowing, such as jumping jacks, running in place, or riding a stationary bike, or to run through at half speed the physical movements to be performed, such as gradually warming up before a tennis match.

The time to perform a good stretching routine is *after* vigorous physical activity, which will fight the body's natural tendency to stiffen up.

Stretching immediately after your abdominal workout assures that the muscles will remain supple and loose and will also help relieve any postworkout soreness. But the five-minute stretch described in this chapter can be performed at any time during the day to relieve accumulated muscular tightness. You will also find these stretching exercises very helpful and relaxing as an early morning wake-up routine or for end-of-the-day stress release.

Stretching should be performed very gently so the muscles won't be injured. To stretch properly, stretch the muscle until you feel tension, then relax. Don't bounce, or make quick or jerky movements, or try to push the muscle past the point of initial tension. Breathe normally, but as you go deeper into a stretch, concentrate on breathing out. Hold each stretch for 20 seconds.

The following exercises are specifically designed to stretch the abdominal muscles, low back muscles, the muscles of the upper and lower leg, and the chest, shoulder, and neck muscles. It should take you five minutes to perform all the stretches outlined here.

1. Iliopsoas Stretch (Front of hip)— Standing Lunge Position

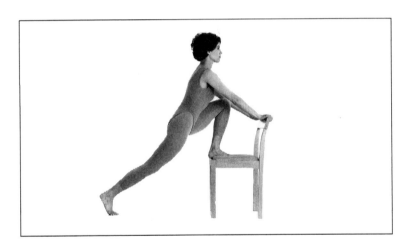

FORM
• Standing, with foot of the hip to be stretched on floor, toes straight ahead, place the other foot on a low table or chair.

EXECUTION
• Lunge forward, raising the heel of the standing leg off the floor.
• Feel the stretch in the front of the hip of the standing leg.
• Hold the stretch 20 seconds.
• Repeat the stretch with the opposite leg.
• Hold the stretch 20 seconds per leg.

Alternative Iliopsoas Stretch—Lunge Position

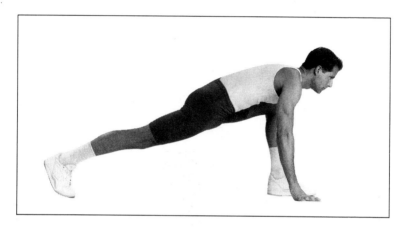

FORM

- Move one leg forward until the knee of the forward leg is directly over the ankle and almost at chest level.
- Keep the back leg straight. Don't drop the rear knee.
- Keep hands shoulder-width apart. Use for balance.
- Look straight ahead as you perform the exercise.

EXECUTION

- Straighten the back leg, placing the weight onto the toes and the ball of the rear foot.
- Do not keep your front knee ahead of your ankle or allow the back knee to bend. This will keep you from stretching properly.
- Think of the front of your hip going down to create stretch tension.
- Hold the stretch for 20 seconds and return to the starting position.
- Repeat with the opposite leg.

2. Quadratus Stretch (Side of lower trunk)

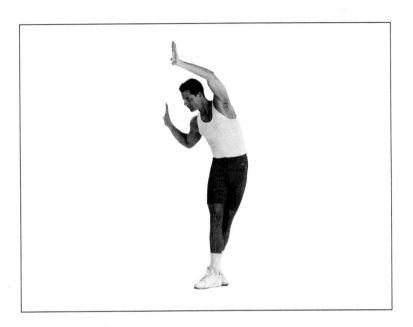

FORM

- Stand sideways to a wall, one foot away, your shoulder sideways to the wall.
- Cross the outside foot behind the other with the weight centered on the ball of that outside foot.
- Place the palm of the hand nearest to the wall against the wall.

EXECUTION

- Swing the opposite arm up and directly over head until it touches the wall, allowing you to side bend. Slightly turn your upper body toward the wall.
- Allow your hips to fall away from the wall.
- Hold this stretch for 20 seconds and repeat on the opposite side.

3. Quadriceps Stretch (Front of thigh)

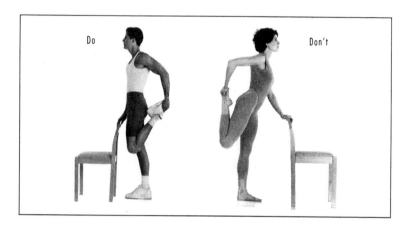

FORM

- Stand facing the back of a chair or a wall with one hand held out for balance and support.
- Bend one knee backward and pull the heel upward toward your buttocks with your hand.

EXECUTION

- Pull your foot gently toward your buttocks.
- Contract your abdominals.
- Hold the stretch for 20 seconds and then repeat with the opposite leg.
- Don't lean too far forward. Make sure back is straight and kept from arching.

4. Seated Hamstring Stretch (Back of thigh)

FORM

- Sit at the edge of a chair or table with back erect.

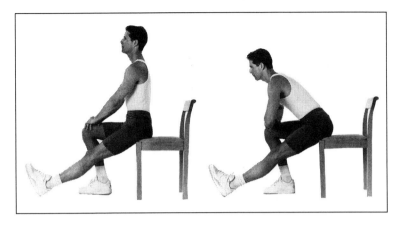

• Extend left leg out in front of you with heel resting on floor.

EXECUTION
• Place palms on upper right thigh.
• Lean gently forward from the hips as far as you can.
• Make sure the heel of the extended leg stays on the floor.
• Hold for 20 seconds. Repeat with the opposite leg.

Alternative Hamstring Stretch

FORM
• Sit on the floor.
• Keep your back straight.
• Extend left leg straight out.
• Place sole of right foot beside extended left thigh.

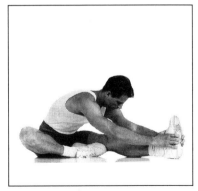

EXECUTION
• Slowly bend forward at the waist and stretch your hands out along your shin until you reach your ankle or toes.
• Hold the stretch for 20 seconds and repeat on the other leg.

5. Seated Buttock-Hip Stretch

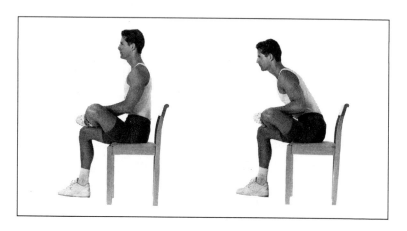

FORM
- Sit at the edge of a chair or table.
- Keep right foot flat on the floor.
- Cross left leg over the right, resting the ankle over your knee.
- Keep hands on the shin of your upper leg.
- Keep your back straight.

EXECUTION
- Gently lean forward from the hips until the stretch is felt at the side of the buttock.
- Hold the stretch for 20 seconds.
- Return to the start position and repeat with the other leg.

Alternative Buttock-Hip Stretch

FORM
- Lie on your back on the mat with knees bent and feet flat on the floor.
- Cross your right leg over the left, resting your right calf muscle just above your left knee.

- Bring your legs toward your chest.
- Intertwine fingers behind left thigh, just below the knee.

EXECUTION

- To stretch the right buttock, gently pull the left knee closer to your chest.
- Hold the stretch for 20 seconds.
- Return to the start position and repeat with the opposite leg.

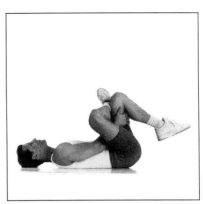

6. Cat/Camel

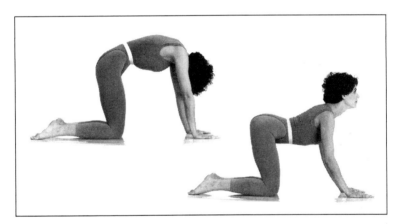

FORM

- Get on the mat on hands and knees with the top of both feet on the floor.
- Look forward.

EXECUTION

- Contract abdominals, and round your back beginning with the lower vertebrae. Keep chin tucked in toward your chest.
- Hold for 10 seconds, relax your abdominals, and return to starting position.

- Arch your back beginning with the lower vertebrae, while at the same time raising your head.
- Hold for 10 seconds.

The six exercises described above are specifically designed to follow your abdominal workout. For a good full-body stretch to be performed in the morning or evening or simply if you are feeling stiff or achy, add the following three exercises.

7. CALF STRETCH

F O R M

Assume the iliopsoas stretch (no. 1) position.

E X E C U T I O N

- Lower your heel to stretch the calf muscle.
- Hold for 20 seconds and repeat with the other leg.

8. CHEST AND SHOULDER STRETCH

F O R M

Stand erect in front of a doorway.
- Place your hands at any level on the door frame.

E X E C U T I O N

- Lean in and step slowly through the doorway, while bending your lead knee slightly.
- Stop when you feel a mild stretch in the chest and shoulders. (May need to raise or lower hands for a better stretch.)
- Hold for 20 seconds.

9. NECK STRETCH

F O R M

Sit up straight in a chair or stand.

E X E C U T I O N

- Lower your left ear toward your left shoulder while simultaneously pulling the right arm down behind your back with your left hand.
- Hold for 20 seconds.
- Repeat on the right side.

7

Low-Fat Eating

To pare away excess body fat overlaying the midsection and make your abdominal muscles stand out, you need to reduce the amount of fatty foods that you eat each day.

Nutrition studies show that when fat-rich foods are consumed they tend to settle all too easily in the abdomen, stored there as body fat. Getting rid of this excess fat is not so easy anymore because modern living, with all of its comforts and technological advances, has radically altered the amount of physical movement in our daily routines.

Thus, it's important that your diet reflect a reality-based approach to nutrition. Most Americans currently eat a diet that is over 40 percent fat, a level most nutrition experts say is at least 10 percent too high. Diets that are saturated with fat are directly linked with heart disease, diabetes, obesity, and other serious health consequences. Therefore, you should strive to reduce fat intake to the 30 percent range or lower. You can take simple measures to limit your daily fat intake by using the new Food Group Pyramid.

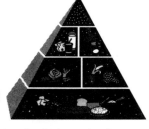

THE FOOD GROUP PYRAMID

By changing your eating habits and eating foods from the Department of Agriculture's newly formulated Food Group Pyramid—which replaces the familiar Food Group Wheel—you will eat less fat but more whole grains, vegetables, and fruits.

At the base of this pyramid are grains (bread, rice, cereal, and pasta). Between 6 and 11 servings a day are recommended. An ounce of dry cereal, ½ cup of cooked rice or pasta, ½ bagel, or 1 slice of bread each constitute a serving from this grain group.

Vegetables and fruits are on the next level, with 3 to 5 servings and 2 to 4 servings respectively recommended daily. A serving of vegetables could be 1 cup of raw, leafy greens or ½ cup of any other vegetable. A banana, orange, or medium apple, or ½ cup of fresh, cooked, or canned fruit, or ¾ cup of fruit juice meets a serving requirement in the fruit group.

As the pyramid narrows, meat, fowl, and fish, along with dairy products—both with a recommended 2 to 3 daily servings—occupy the next level. A cup of milk, 8 ounces of yogurt, or 2 ounces of processed cheese can make a serving in the dairy group, while a daily maximum of 7 ounces of cooked lean meat, fish, or poultry makes a serving in the meat group. Beans (½ cup), 1 egg, and peanut butter (2 tablespoons) count as 1 ounce of meat.

Fats, oils, and sweets are at the very top of the food pyramid, and come with a recommendation to eat them sparingly.

TIPS FOR HEALTHFUL EATING

Most Americans know that they should reduce the amount of fat that they consume daily, but they don't know how. Use the following tips to help you cut back on fats at breakfast, lunch, and dinner.

BREAKFAST

Breakfast is the most important meal of the day. Research shows that if you skip breakfast because you aren't hungry or don't have time to eat, you will pay for it later with energy shortages, concentration lapses, and changes in temperament.

Breakfast doesn't have to be an elaborate sit-down, cooked affair, but can be as simple as a bran muffin, yogurt, and a banana. Here are some quick, nutritious breakfasts that require little prep time, as well as some tips for reducing fats.

- An English muffin, bran muffin, bagel, or slice of grain toast. Skip the croissant or pastry, both of which are high-fat.
- A high-fiber cereal with 4 grams of fiber and less than 5 grams of fat. Check the cereal box label for nutritional content.
- When choosing a juice, be sure fruit juice is 100 percent juice and not juice "beverage" made with added water and sugar.
- Yogurt with bran or granola sprinkled on top. If sprinkling granola on your cereal or yogurt, use your own homemade variety. Excessive amounts of saturated fats and coconut oil are used in many store-bought varieties.
- A bagel with a light coating of cream cheese and a glass of juice.
- A banana with a glass of skim or low-fat milk.
- A bowl of iron-enriched cereal, low-fat milk, and a sliced banana.
- To reduce the amount of cholesterol in your diet, limit yourself to three eggs per week.
- Reduce the amount of bacon you eat, or replace it with Canadian bacon, which has less fat.
- Eliminate whole milk from the diet and switch to 2 percent milk, eventually going to 1 percent, finally to skim milk.

LUNCH

Sandwiches provide the staple for the American lunchtime diet, but since most luncheon meats are high in fat content, try turkey, chicken, or tuna with a side order of green salad. Vinegar and olive oil dressing or one with lemon juice is much better than salad dressing made with fat-laden mayonnaise.

A few slices of pizza and some fruit juice make a fine lunch. If you want to eat at your desk, bring in a box of low-fat crackers, some peanut butter, and a piece of fruit and you'll have all that you need for a quick, hearty meal.

DINNER

Most people consider dinner to be the main meal of the day. You need to pay close attention here or you can easily tip the fat scales very quickly with meats and fat-rich sauces. If you've eaten carefully during the day, this meal doesn't have to be packed with calories or require tremendous preparation. Use the following tips to help prepare delicious, low-fat, satisfying dinners.

- Begin your meal with a broth-based soup or green salad. These low-fat dinner items will cut your appetite and you will end up eating less meat for your main course.
- Replace your meat course with fish or poultry several times a week. Skinless poultry has less fat than red meat.
- Think pasta.
- In place of high-fat sauces or butter on your vegetables, try yogurt dressing, herbs, or lemon juice. These no-fat alternatives are tasty and quite satisfying.
- In recipes that call for milk, butter, or cream, substitute vegetable or chicken broth whenever appropriate.

PLAN AHEAD

If you continually have a hectic schedule throughout the week, it's best to set aside some time on the weekend to prepare food for the upcoming week. It may seem tedious to spend time washing, cleaning, and slicing fruit and vegetables and putting them in plastic containers in the refrigerator, but this way there will always be something low-fat readily available to eat throughout the week.

- In addition to carrots, celery, and fruit, other food items that can be prepared ahead of time include low-fat cheese, cubed or cut into small portions. Pizzas, made on English muffins and either frozen or refrigerated, also make great snacks or a light meal.
- If your favorite fruit is currently out of season, substitute a canned variety. Canned fruit makes a wholesome snack with little difference in nutritional value when compared to fresh or frozen fruit. If the fruit is packed in a heavy, sugar-based syrup, drain it so you won't take in empty sugar calories.
- For more substantial meals that require little daily preparation, cook a lean roast beef or turkey on the weekend. This can then be consumed throughout the week at different meals.
- Always have on hand a varied selection of frozen vegetables such as broccoli and spinach, or potatoes that can be boiled or put in the microwave. Then nutritious meals high in carbohydrates and low in fats can be ready in an instant.

STOCKING THE CUPBOARD

You can easily pull together a low-fat, no-cook meal or quickly prepare a hot dinner when you have basic foodstuffs available at home.
Standard dinner fare can be as simple as English muffin pizzas; stoned
wheat crackers, peanut butter, and milk; vegetable soup with extra
broccoli and a sprinkling of Parmesan cheese; tuna sandwich with
tomato soup; or bran cereal with banana and raisins.
Keep the following items on hand:

CUPBOARD

Spaghetti
Rice
Potatoes
Wheat crackers
Spaghetti sauce
Minced clams
Tuna

Canned salmon
Kidney beans
Peanut butter
Bran flakes
Oat bran
Raisins

REFRIGERATOR

"Lite" cheese
Parmesan cheese
Low-fat cottage cheese
Low-fat yogurt
Low-fat milk

Eggs
Bananas and a variety of other
    fruits
Carrots

FREEZER

English muffins
Pita bread
Multigrain bread
Orange juice concentrate
Broccoli

Spinach
Winter squash
Cut-up chicken
Extra-lean hamburger
Ground turkey

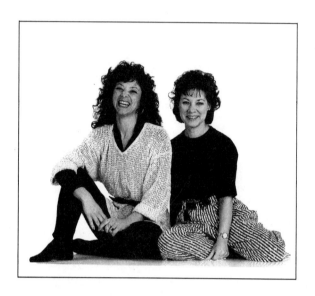

Jeanette Micelotta, M.S., P.T., is the Chief Physical Therapist at the Center for Sports and Osteopathic Medicine in New York City.
Deborah Michaels, P.T.A., is a Practicing Physical Therapist at the Center for Sports and Osteopathic Medicine.